THIS BOOK BELONGS TO:

CONTACT INFORMATION	
NAME:	
ADDRESS:	
PHONE:	

START / END DATES

_____ / _____ / _____   TO   _____ / _____ / _____

DEDICATION

This Headache Journal Log book is dedicated to all the headache sufferers out there who want to record their headaches and document their findings in the process.

You are my inspiration for producing books and I'm honored to be a part of keeping all of your Headache notes and records organized.

This journal, notebook will help you record your details about your headaches.

Thoughtfully put together with these sections to record:

Date, Start & End Time, Duration, Severity of Headache, Location, Triggers, Details, Weather, Other Symptoms, Relief Solutions, Medication, Other, and Notes.

HOW TO USE THIS BOOK

The purpose of this book is to keep all of your Headache notes all in one place. It will help keep you organized.

This Headache Journal will allow you to accurately document every detail about your headaches. It's a great way to chart your course through managing your headaches.

Here are examples of the prompts for you to fill in and write about your experience in this book:

1. **Date** - Write the date.
2. **Start & End Time** - Record the start and end time of your headache or migraine.
3. **Duration** - Log how long your headache last.
4. **Severity Of Headache** - Rate your level of pain from 0-10.
5. **Location** - Where your headache is located.
6. **Triggers, Details** - What activity, if any, were you doing. Any smells, were you outside in the sun, etc.
7. **Weather** - What was the weather like outside, sinus season, etc.
8. **Other Symptoms** - Record any other symptoms you may be having.
9. **Relief Solutions** - If you were able to get relief, what treatment worked, sleep it off, the food you ate, or water intake.
10. **Medication** - Log what medications you are taking.
11. **Other** - Write any other information you don't want to forget.
12. **Notes** - Record any other important information, daily headaches, best pain management you've found that works.

Headache Log

DATE	TIME STARTED
DURATION	TIME ENDED

Severity of headache

0	1	2	3	4	5	6	7	8	9	10

LOCATION	WEATHER
	OTHER SYMPTOMS

Triggers

DETAILS

Relief solutions

MEDICATION

OTHER

NOTES

Headache Log

DATE	TIME STARTED
DURATION	TIME ENDED

Severity of headache

0	1	2	3	4	5	6	7	8	9	10

LOCATION	WEATHER
	OTHER SYMPTOMS

Triggers

DETAILS

Relief solutions

MEDICATION

OTHER

NOTES

HEADACHE LOG

DATE	TIME STARTED
DURATION	TIME ENDED

SEVERITY OF HEADACHE

0 1 2 3 4 5 6 7 8 9 10

LOCATION	WEATHER
	OTHER SYMPTOMS

TRIGGERS

DETAILS

RELIEF SOLUTIONS

MEDICATION

OTHER

NOTES

Headache Log

Date	Time started
Duration	Time ended

Severity of headache

0	1	2	3	4	5	6	7	8	9	10

Location	Weather
	Other symptoms

Triggers

Details

Relief solutions

Medication

Other

Notes

Headache Log

DATE	TIME STARTED
DURATION	TIME ENDED

Severity of headache

0	1	2	3	4	5	6	7	8	9	10

LOCATION	WEATHER
	OTHER SYMPTOMS

Triggers

DETAILS

Relief solutions

MEDICATION

OTHER

NOTES

Headache Log

DATE	TIME STARTED
DURATION	TIME ENDED

Severity of headache

| 0 | 1 | 2 | 3 | 4 | 5 | 6 | 7 | 8 | 9 | 10 |

LOCATION	WEATHER
	OTHER SYMPTOMS

Triggers

DETAILS

Relief solutions

MEDICATION

OTHER

NOTES

Headache Log

DATE	TIME STARTED
DURATION	**TIME ENDED**

Severity of headache

0	1	2	3	4	5	6	7	8	9	10

LOCATION	WEATHER
	OTHER SYMPTOMS

Triggers

DETAILS

Relief solutions

MEDICATION

OTHER

NOTES

HEADACHE LOG

DATE	TIME STARTED
DURATION	TIME ENDED

SEVERITY OF HEADACHE

0	1	2	3	4	5	6	7	8	9	10

LOCATION	WEATHER
	OTHER SYMPTOMS

TRIGGERS

DETAILS

RELIEF SOLUTIONS

MEDICATION

OTHER

NOTES

Headache Log

DATE	TIME STARTED
DURATION	TIME ENDED

Severity of headache

0 1 2 3 4 5 6 7 8 9 10

LOCATION	WEATHER
	OTHER SYMPTOMS

Triggers

DETAILS

Relief solutions

MEDICATION

OTHER

NOTES

Headache Log

DATE	TIME STARTED
DURATION	TIME ENDED

Severity of headache

0	1	2	3	4	5	6	7	8	9	10

LOCATION	WEATHER
	OTHER SYMPTOMS

Triggers

DETAILS

Relief solutions

MEDICATION

OTHER

NOTES

Headache Log

DATE	TIME STARTED
DURATION	TIME ENDED

Severity of headache

| 0 | 1 | 2 | 3 | 4 | 5 | 6 | 7 | 8 | 9 | 10 |

LOCATION	WEATHER
	OTHER SYMPTOMS

Triggers

DETAILS

Relief solutions

MEDICATION

OTHER

NOTES

Headache Log

DATE	TIME STARTED
DURATION	TIME ENDED

Severity of headache

0	1	2	3	4	5	6	7	8	9	10

LOCATION	WEATHER
	OTHER SYMPTOMS

Triggers

DETAILS

Relief solutions

MEDICATION

OTHER

NOTES

HEADACHE LOG

DATE	TIME STARTED
DURATION	TIME ENDED

SEVERITY OF HEADACHE

0	1	2	3	4	5	6	7	8	9	10

LOCATION	WEATHER
	OTHER SYMPTOMS

TRIGGERS

DETAILS

RELIEF SOLUTIONS

MEDICATION

OTHER

NOTES

Headache Log

DATE	TIME STARTED
DURATION	TIME ENDED

Severity of headache

0	1	2	3	4	5	6	7	8	9	10

LOCATION	WEATHER
	OTHER SYMPTOMS

Triggers

DETAILS

Relief solutions

MEDICATION

OTHER

NOTES

Headache Log

DATE	TIME STARTED
DURATION	TIME ENDED

Severity of headache

0	1	2	3	4	5	6	7	8	9	10

LOCATION	WEATHER
	OTHER SYMPTOMS

Triggers

DETAILS

Relief solutions

MEDICATION

OTHER

NOTES

Headache Log

DATE	TIME STARTED
DURATION	TIME ENDED

SEVERITY OF HEADACHE

0   1   2   3   4   5   6   7   8   9   10

LOCATION	WEATHER
	OTHER SYMPTOMS

TRIGGERS

DETAILS

RELIEF SOLUTIONS

MEDICATION

OTHER

NOTES

Headache Log

DATE	TIME STARTED
DURATION	TIME ENDED

SEVERITY OF HEADACHE

0 1 2 3 4 5 6 7 8 9 10

LOCATION	WEATHER
	OTHER SYMPTOMS

TRIGGERS

DETAILS

RELIEF SOLUTIONS

MEDICATION

OTHER

NOTES

Headache Log

DATE	TIME STARTED
DURATION	TIME ENDED

Severity of headache

0	1	2	3	4	5	6	7	8	9	10

LOCATION	WEATHER
	OTHER SYMPTOMS

Triggers

DETAILS

Relief solutions

MEDICATION

OTHER

NOTES

Headache Log

DATE	TIME STARTED
DURATION	TIME ENDED

Severity of headache

0	1	2	3	4	5	6	7	8	9	10

LOCATION	WEATHER
	OTHER SYMPTOMS

Triggers

DETAILS

Relief solutions

MEDICATION

OTHER

NOTES

Headache Log

DATE	TIME STARTED
DURATION	TIME ENDED

Severity of headache

0	1	2	3	4	5	6	7	8	9	10

LOCATION	WEATHER
	OTHER SYMPTOMS

Triggers

DETAILS

Relief solutions

MEDICATION

OTHER

NOTES

Headache Log

DATE	TIME STARTED
DURATION	TIME ENDED

Severity of headache

0	1	2	3	4	5	6	7	8	9	10

LOCATION	WEATHER
	OTHER SYMPTOMS

Triggers

DETAILS

Relief solutions

MEDICATION

OTHER

NOTES

Headache Log

DATE	TIME STARTED
DURATION	TIME ENDED

Severity of headache

0   1   2   3   4   5   6   7   8   9   10

LOCATION	WEATHER
	OTHER SYMPTOMS

Triggers

DETAILS

Relief solutions

MEDICATION

OTHER

NOTES

Headache Log

DATE	TIME STARTED
DURATION	TIME ENDED

Severity of headache

0	1	2	3	4	5	6	7	8	9	10

LOCATION	WEATHER
	OTHER SYMPTOMS

Triggers

DETAILS

Relief solutions

MEDICATION

OTHER

NOTES

Headache Log

DATE	TIME STARTED
DURATION	TIME ENDED

Severity of headache

0	1	2	3	4	5	6	7	8	9	10

LOCATION	WEATHER
	OTHER SYMPTOMS

Triggers

DETAILS

Relief solutions

MEDICATION

OTHER

NOTES

Headache Log

DATE	TIME STARTED
DURATION	TIME ENDED

Severity of headache

0	1	2	3	4	5	6	7	8	9	10

LOCATION	WEATHER
	OTHER SYMPTOMS

Triggers

DETAILS

Relief solutions

MEDICATION

OTHER

NOTES

Headache Log

DATE	TIME STARTED
DURATION	**TIME ENDED**

Severity of headache

0   1   2   3   4   5   6   7   8   9   10

LOCATION	WEATHER
	OTHER SYMPTOMS

Triggers

DETAILS

Relief solutions

MEDICATION

OTHER

NOTES

Headache Log

DATE	TIME STARTED
DURATION	TIME ENDED

Severity of headache

0	1	2	3	4	5	6	7	8	9	10

LOCATION	WEATHER
	OTHER SYMPTOMS

Triggers

DETAILS

Relief solutions

MEDICATION

OTHER

NOTES

HEADACHE LOG

DATE	TIME STARTED
DURATION	TIME ENDED

SEVERITY OF HEADACHE

0 1 2 3 4 5 6 7 8 9 10

LOCATION	WEATHER
	OTHER SYMPTOMS

TRIGGERS

DETAILS

RELIEF SOLUTIONS

MEDICATION

OTHER

NOTES

Headache Log

DATE	TIME STARTED
DURATION	TIME ENDED

Severity of headache

0	1	2	3	4	5	6	7	8	9	10

LOCATION	WEATHER
	OTHER SYMPTOMS

Triggers

DETAILS

Relief solutions

MEDICATION

OTHER

NOTES

Headache Log

DATE	TIME STARTED
DURATION	TIME ENDED

Severity of headache

0	1	2	3	4	5	6	7	8	9	10

LOCATION	WEATHER
	OTHER SYMPTOMS

Triggers

DETAILS

Relief solutions

MEDICATION

OTHER

NOTES

Headache Log

DATE	TIME STARTED
DURATION	TIME ENDED

Severity of headache

0	1	2	3	4	5	6	7	8	9	10

LOCATION	WEATHER
	OTHER SYMPTOMS

Triggers

DETAILS

Relief solutions

MEDICATION

OTHER

NOTES

Headache Log

DATE	TIME STARTED
DURATION	TIME ENDED

Severity of headache

0	1	2	3	4	5	6	7	8	9	10

LOCATION	WEATHER
	OTHER SYMPTOMS

Triggers

DETAILS

Relief solutions

MEDICATION

OTHER

NOTES

Headache Log

DATE	TIME STARTED
DURATION	TIME ENDED

Severity of headache

0	1	2	3	4	5	6	7	8	9	10

LOCATION	WEATHER
	OTHER SYMPTOMS

Triggers

DETAILS

Relief solutions

MEDICATION

OTHER

NOTES

Headache Log

DATE	TIME STARTED
DURATION	TIME ENDED

Severity of headache

0	1	2	3	4	5	6	7	8	9	10

LOCATION	WEATHER
	OTHER SYMPTOMS

Triggers

DETAILS

Relief solutions

MEDICATION

OTHER

NOTES

Headache Log

DATE	TIME STARTED
DURATION	TIME ENDED

Severity of headache

0 1 2 3 4 5 6 7 8 9 10

LOCATION	WEATHER
	OTHER SYMPTOMS

Triggers

DETAILS

Relief solutions

MEDICATION

OTHER

NOTES

Headache Log

DATE	TIME STARTED
DURATION	TIME ENDED

Severity of headache

0	1	2	3	4	5	6	7	8	9	10

LOCATION	WEATHER
	OTHER SYMPTOMS

Triggers

DETAILS

Relief solutions

MEDICATION

OTHER

NOTES

Headache Log

DATE	TIME STARTED
DURATION	**TIME ENDED**

Severity of headache

| 0 | 1 | 2 | 3 | 4 | 5 | 6 | 7 | 8 | 9 | 10 |

LOCATION	WEATHER
	OTHER SYMPTOMS

Triggers

DETAILS

Relief solutions

MEDICATION

OTHER

NOTES

HEADACHE LOG

DATE	TIME STARTED
DURATION	TIME ENDED

SEVERITY OF HEADACHE

0	1	2	3	4	5	6	7	8	9	10

LOCATION	WEATHER
	OTHER SYMPTOMS

TRIGGERS

DETAILS

RELIEF SOLUTIONS

MEDICATION

OTHER

NOTES

Headache Log

DATE	TIME STARTED
DURATION	TIME ENDED

Severity of headache

0	1	2	3	4	5	6	7	8	9	10

LOCATION	WEATHER
	OTHER SYMPTOMS

Triggers

DETAILS

Relief solutions

MEDICATION

OTHER

NOTES

Headache Log

DATE	TIME STARTED
DURATION	TIME ENDED

Severity of headache

0   1   2   3   4   5   6   7   8   9   10

LOCATION	WEATHER
	OTHER SYMPTOMS

Triggers

DETAILS

Relief solutions

MEDICATION

OTHER

NOTES

Headache Log

DATE	TIME STARTED
DURATION	TIME ENDED

Severity of headache

0	1	2	3	4	5	6	7	8	9	10

LOCATION	WEATHER
	OTHER SYMPTOMS

Triggers

DETAILS

Relief solutions

MEDICATION

OTHER

NOTES

HEADACHE LOG

DATE	TIME STARTED
DURATION	**TIME ENDED**

SEVERITY OF HEADACHE

0	1	2	3	4	5	6	7	8	9	10

LOCATION	WEATHER
	OTHER SYMPTOMS

TRIGGERS

DETAILS

RELIEF SOLUTIONS

MEDICATION

OTHER

NOTES

Headache Log

DATE	TIME STARTED
DURATION	TIME ENDED

Severity of headache

0	1	2	3	4	5	6	7	8	9	10

LOCATION	WEATHER
	OTHER SYMPTOMS

Triggers

DETAILS

Relief solutions

MEDICATION

OTHER

NOTES

Headache Log

DATE	TIME STARTED
DURATION	**TIME ENDED**

Severity of headache

| 0 | 1 | 2 | 3 | 4 | 5 | 6 | 7 | 8 | 9 | 10 |

LOCATION	WEATHER
	OTHER SYMPTOMS

Triggers

DETAILS

Relief solutions

MEDICATION

OTHER

NOTES

HEADACHE LOG

DATE	TIME STARTED
DURATION	TIME ENDED

SEVERITY OF HEADACHE

| 0 | 1 | 2 | 3 | 4 | 5 | 6 | 7 | 8 | 9 | 10 |

LOCATION	WEATHER
	OTHER SYMPTOMS

TRIGGERS

DETAILS

RELIEF SOLUTIONS

MEDICATION

OTHER

NOTES

Headache Log

DATE	TIME STARTED
DURATION	TIME ENDED

SEVERITY OF HEADACHE

0	1	2	3	4	5	6	7	8	9	10

LOCATION	WEATHER
	OTHER SYMPTOMS

TRIGGERS

DETAILS

RELIEF SOLUTIONS

MEDICATION

OTHER

NOTES

Headache Log

DATE	TIME STARTED
DURATION	TIME ENDED

Severity of headache

0	1	2	3	4	5	6	7	8	9	10

LOCATION	WEATHER
	OTHER SYMPTOMS

Triggers

DETAILS

Relief solutions

MEDICATION

OTHER

NOTES

Headache Log

DATE	TIME STARTED
DURATION	TIME ENDED

Severity of headache

0	1	2	3	4	5	6	7	8	9	10

LOCATION	WEATHER
	OTHER SYMPTOMS

Triggers

DETAILS

Relief solutions

MEDICATION

OTHER

NOTES

HEADACHE LOG

DATE	TIME STARTED
DURATION	TIME ENDED

SEVERITY OF HEADACHE

0   1   2   3   4   5   6   7   8   9   10

LOCATION	WEATHER
	OTHER SYMPTOMS

TRIGGERS

DETAILS

RELIEF SOLUTIONS

MEDICATION

OTHER

NOTES

HEADACHE LOG

DATE	TIME STARTED
DURATION	**TIME ENDED**

SEVERITY OF HEADACHE

0	1	2	3	4	5	6	7	8	9	10

LOCATION	WEATHER
	OTHER SYMPTOMS

TRIGGERS

DETAILS

RELIEF SOLUTIONS

MEDICATION

OTHER

NOTES

Headache Log

DATE	TIME STARTED
DURATION	TIME ENDED

Severity of headache

0	1	2	3	4	5	6	7	8	9	10

LOCATION	WEATHER
	OTHER SYMPTOMS

Triggers

DETAILS

Relief solutions

MEDICATION

OTHER

NOTES

Headache Log

DATE	TIME STARTED
DURATION	TIME ENDED

Severity of headache

0	1	2	3	4	5	6	7	8	9	10

LOCATION	WEATHER
	OTHER SYMPTOMS

Triggers

DETAILS

Relief solutions

MEDICATION

OTHER

NOTES

Headache Log

DATE	TIME STARTED
DURATION	TIME ENDED

Severity of headache

| 0 | 1 | 2 | 3 | 4 | 5 | 6 | 7 | 8 | 9 | 10 |

LOCATION

WEATHER

OTHER SYMPTOMS

Triggers

DETAILS

Relief solutions

MEDICATION

OTHER

NOTES

Headache Log

DATE	TIME STARTED
DURATION	TIME ENDED

SEVERITY OF HEADACHE

0   1   2   3   4   5   6   7   8   9   10

LOCATION	WEATHER
	OTHER SYMPTOMS

TRIGGERS

DETAILS

RELIEF SOLUTIONS

MEDICATION

OTHER

NOTES

HEADACHE LOG

DATE	TIME STARTED
DURATION	TIME ENDED

SEVERITY OF HEADACHE

0   1   2   3   4   5   6   7   8   9   10

LOCATION	WEATHER
	OTHER SYMPTOMS

TRIGGERS

DETAILS

RELIEF SOLUTIONS

MEDICATION

OTHER

NOTES

Headache Log

Date	Time started
Duration	Time ended

Severity of headache

0	1	2	3	4	5	6	7	8	9	10

Location	Weather
	Other symptoms

Triggers

Details

Relief solutions

Medication

Other

Notes

Headache Log

Date	Time started
Duration	**Time ended**

Severity of headache

0	1	2	3	4	5	6	7	8	9	10

Location	Weather
	Other symptoms

Triggers

Details

Relief solutions

Medication

Other

Notes

Headache Log

DATE	TIME STARTED
DURATION	TIME ENDED

Severity of headache

0　1　2　3　4　5　6　7　8　9　10

LOCATION	WEATHER
	OTHER SYMPTOMS

Triggers

DETAILS

Relief solutions

MEDICATION

OTHER

NOTES

Headache Log

DATE	TIME STARTED
DURATION	TIME ENDED

Severity of headache

0	1	2	3	4	5	6	7	8	9	10

LOCATION	WEATHER
	OTHER SYMPTOMS

Triggers

DETAILS

Relief solutions

MEDICATION

OTHER

NOTES

Headache Log

DATE	TIME STARTED
DURATION	**TIME ENDED**

Severity of headache

0 1 2 3 4 5 6 7 8 9 10

LOCATION	WEATHER
	OTHER SYMPTOMS

Triggers

DETAILS

Relief solutions

MEDICATION

OTHER

NOTES

Headache Log

DATE	TIME STARTED
DURATION	TIME ENDED

Severity of headache

0	1	2	3	4	5	6	7	8	9	10

LOCATION	WEATHER
	OTHER SYMPTOMS

Triggers

DETAILS

Relief solutions

MEDICATION

OTHER

NOTES

Headache Log

DATE	TIME STARTED
DURATION	TIME ENDED

Severity of headache

0	1	2	3	4	5	6	7	8	9	10

LOCATION	WEATHER
	OTHER SYMPTOMS

Triggers

DETAILS

Relief solutions

MEDICATION

OTHER

NOTES

Headache Log

DATE	TIME STARTED
DURATION	TIME ENDED

Severity of Headache

0 1 2 3 4 5 6 7 8 9 10

LOCATION	WEATHER
	OTHER SYMPTOMS

Triggers

DETAILS

Relief Solutions

MEDICATION

OTHER

NOTES

Headache Log

DATE	TIME STARTED
DURATION	TIME ENDED

SEVERITY OF HEADACHE

0	1	2	3	4	5	6	7	8	9	10

LOCATION	WEATHER
	OTHER SYMPTOMS

TRIGGERS

DETAILS

RELIEF SOLUTIONS

MEDICATION

OTHER

NOTES

HEADACHE LOG

DATE	TIME STARTED
DURATION	TIME ENDED

SEVERITY OF HEADACHE

0	1	2	3	4	5	6	7	8	9	10

LOCATION	WEATHER
	OTHER SYMPTOMS

TRIGGERS

DETAILS

RELIEF SOLUTIONS

MEDICATION

OTHER

NOTES

Headache Log

DATE	TIME STARTED
DURATION	TIME ENDED

Severity of headache

0 1 2 3 4 5 6 7 8 9 10

LOCATION	WEATHER
	OTHER SYMPTOMS

Triggers

DETAILS

Relief solutions

MEDICATION

OTHER

NOTES

Headache Log

DATE	TIME STARTED
DURATION	TIME ENDED

Severity of headache

0	1	2	3	4	5	6	7	8	9	10

LOCATION	WEATHER
	OTHER SYMPTOMS

Triggers

DETAILS

Relief solutions

MEDICATION

OTHER

NOTES

Headache Log

DATE	TIME STARTED
DURATION	TIME ENDED

Severity of headache

| 0 | 1 | 2 | 3 | 4 | 5 | 6 | 7 | 8 | 9 | 10 |

LOCATION	WEATHER
	OTHER SYMPTOMS

Triggers

DETAILS

Relief solutions

MEDICATION

OTHER

NOTES

HEADACHE LOG

DATE	TIME STARTED
DURATION	TIME ENDED

SEVERITY OF HEADACHE

0	1	2	3	4	5	6	7	8	9	10

LOCATION	WEATHER
	OTHER SYMPTOMS

TRIGGERS

DETAILS

RELIEF SOLUTIONS

MEDICATION

OTHER

NOTES

Headache Log

DATE	TIME STARTED
DURATION	TIME ENDED

SEVERITY OF HEADACHE

| 0 | 1 | 2 | 3 | 4 | 5 | 6 | 7 | 8 | 9 | 10 |

LOCATION	WEATHER
	OTHER SYMPTOMS

TRIGGERS

DETAILS

RELIEF SOLUTIONS

MEDICATION

OTHER

NOTES

Headache Log

DATE	TIME STARTED
DURATION	TIME ENDED

Severity of headache

0	1	2	3	4	5	6	7	8	9	10

LOCATION	WEATHER
	OTHER SYMPTOMS

Triggers

DETAILS

Relief solutions

MEDICATION

OTHER

NOTES

Headache Log

DATE	TIME STARTED
DURATION	TIME ENDED

Severity of headache

| 0 | 1 | 2 | 3 | 4 | 5 | 6 | 7 | 8 | 9 | 10 |

LOCATION	WEATHER
	OTHER SYMPTOMS

Triggers

DETAILS

Relief solutions

MEDICATION

OTHER

NOTES

Headache Log

DATE	TIME STARTED
DURATION	TIME ENDED

Severity of headache

0   1   2   3   4   5   6   7   8   9   10

LOCATION	WEATHER
	OTHER SYMPTOMS

Triggers

DETAILS

Relief solutions

MEDICATION

OTHER

NOTES

Headache Log

DATE	TIME STARTED
DURATION	TIME ENDED

Severity of headache

0	1	2	3	4	5	6	7	8	9	10

LOCATION	WEATHER
	OTHER SYMPTOMS

Triggers

DETAILS

Relief solutions

MEDICATION

OTHER

NOTES

Headache Log

DATE	TIME STARTED
DURATION	TIME ENDED

Severity of headache

| 0 | 1 | 2 | 3 | 4 | 5 | 6 | 7 | 8 | 9 | 10 |

LOCATION	WEATHER
	OTHER SYMPTOMS

Triggers

DETAILS

Relief solutions

MEDICATION

OTHER

NOTES

Headache Log

DATE	TIME STARTED
DURATION	TIME ENDED

Severity of headache

0	1	2	3	4	5	6	7	8	9	10

LOCATION	WEATHER
	OTHER SYMPTOMS

Triggers

DETAILS

Relief solutions

MEDICATION

OTHER

NOTES

Headache Log

DATE	TIME STARTED
DURATION	TIME ENDED

Severity of headache

0 1 2 3 4 5 6 7 8 9 10

LOCATION	WEATHER
	OTHER SYMPTOMS

Triggers

DETAILS

Relief solutions

MEDICATION

OTHER

NOTES

Headache Log

DATE	TIME STARTED
DURATION	**TIME ENDED**

Severity of headache

0   1   2   3   4   5   6   7   8   9   10

LOCATION	WEATHER
	OTHER SYMPTOMS

Triggers

DETAILS

Relief solutions

MEDICATION

OTHER

NOTES

HEADACHE LOG

DATE	TIME STARTED
DURATION	TIME ENDED

SEVERITY OF HEADACHE

0   1   2   3   4   5   6   7   8   9   10

LOCATION	WEATHER
	OTHER SYMPTOMS

TRIGGERS

DETAILS

RELIEF SOLUTIONS

MEDICATION

OTHER

NOTES

Headache Log

DATE	TIME STARTED
DURATION	TIME ENDED

Severity of headache

0	1	2	3	4	5	6	7	8	9	10

LOCATION	WEATHER
	OTHER SYMPTOMS

Triggers

DETAILS

Relief solutions

MEDICATION

OTHER

NOTES

Headache Log

DATE	TIME STARTED
DURATION	TIME ENDED

Severity of headache

0	1	2	3	4	5	6	7	8	9	10

LOCATION	WEATHER
	OTHER SYMPTOMS

Triggers

DETAILS

Relief solutions

MEDICATION

OTHER

NOTES

Headache Log

DATE	TIME STARTED
DURATION	TIME ENDED

SEVERITY OF HEADACHE

0	1	2	3	4	5	6	7	8	9	10

LOCATION	WEATHER
	OTHER SYMPTOMS

TRIGGERS

DETAILS

RELIEF SOLUTIONS

MEDICATION

OTHER

NOTES

Headache Log

Date	Time started
Duration	Time ended

Severity of headache

0	1	2	3	4	5	6	7	8	9	10

Location	Weather
	Other symptoms

Triggers

Details

Relief solutions

Medication

Other

Notes

Headache Log

DATE	TIME STARTED
DURATION	**TIME ENDED**

Severity of headache

0 1 2 3 4 5 6 7 8 9 10

LOCATION	WEATHER
	OTHER SYMPTOMS

Triggers

DETAILS

Relief solutions

MEDICATION

OTHER

NOTES

Headache Log

DATE	TIME STARTED
DURATION	TIME ENDED

Severity of headache

| 0 | 1 | 2 | 3 | 4 | 5 | 6 | 7 | 8 | 9 | 10 |

LOCATION	WEATHER
	OTHER SYMPTOMS

Triggers

DETAILS

Relief solutions

MEDICATION

OTHER

NOTES

Headache Log

Date	Time started
Duration	Time ended

Severity of headache

0	1	2	3	4	5	6	7	8	9	10

Location	Weather
	Other symptoms

Triggers

Details

Relief solutions

Medication

Other

Notes

Headache Log

DATE	TIME STARTED
DURATION	TIME ENDED

Severity of headache

0	1	2	3	4	5	6	7	8	9	10

LOCATION	WEATHER
	OTHER SYMPTOMS

Triggers

DETAILS

Relief solutions

MEDICATION

OTHER

NOTES

Headache Log

DATE	TIME STARTED
DURATION	TIME ENDED

Severity of headache

0   1   2   3   4   5   6   7   8   9   10

LOCATION	WEATHER
	OTHER SYMPTOMS

Triggers

DETAILS

Relief solutions

MEDICATION

OTHER

NOTES

Headache Log

DATE	TIME STARTED
DURATION	TIME ENDED

Severity of headache

0	1	2	3	4	5	6	7	8	9	10

LOCATION	WEATHER
	OTHER SYMPTOMS

Triggers

DETAILS

Relief solutions

MEDICATION

OTHER

NOTES

Headache Log

DATE	TIME STARTED
DURATION	TIME ENDED

SEVERITY OF HEADACHE

0	1	2	3	4	5	6	7	8	9	10

LOCATION	WEATHER
	OTHER SYMPTOMS

TRIGGERS

DETAILS

RELIEF SOLUTIONS

MEDICATION

OTHER

NOTES

Headache Log

DATE	TIME STARTED
DURATION	TIME ENDED

SEVERITY OF HEADACHE

0 1 2 3 4 5 6 7 8 9 10

LOCATION	WEATHER
	OTHER SYMPTOMS

TRIGGERS

DETAILS

RELIEF SOLUTIONS

MEDICATION

OTHER

NOTES

HEADACHE LOG

DATE	TIME STARTED
DURATION	TIME ENDED

SEVERITY OF HEADACHE

0   1   2   3   4   5   6   7   8   9   10

LOCATION	WEATHER
	OTHER SYMPTOMS

TRIGGERS

DETAILS

RELIEF SOLUTIONS

MEDICATION

OTHER

NOTES

Headache Log

DATE	**TIME STARTED**
DURATION	**TIME ENDED**

Severity of headache

0	1	2	3	4	5	6	7	8	9	10

LOCATION	**WEATHER**
	OTHER SYMPTOMS

Triggers

DETAILS

Relief solutions

MEDICATION

OTHER

NOTES

Headache Log

DATE	TIME STARTED
DURATION	TIME ENDED

Severity of headache

0	1	2	3	4	5	6	7	8	9	10

LOCATION	WEATHER
	OTHER SYMPTOMS

Triggers

DETAILS

Relief solutions

MEDICATION

OTHER

NOTES

HEADACHE LOG

DATE	TIME STARTED
DURATION	TIME ENDED

SEVERITY OF HEADACHE

0 1 2 3 4 5 6 7 8 9 10

LOCATION	WEATHER
	OTHER SYMPTOMS

TRIGGERS

DETAILS

RELIEF SOLUTIONS

MEDICATION

OTHER

NOTES

Headache Log

DATE	TIME STARTED
DURATION	TIME ENDED

SEVERITY OF HEADACHE

0	1	2	3	4	5	6	7	8	9	10

LOCATION	WEATHER
	OTHER SYMPTOMS

TRIGGERS

DETAILS

RELIEF SOLUTIONS

MEDICATION

OTHER

NOTES

Headache Log

Date	**Time started**
Duration	**Time ended**

Severity of headache

0	1	2	3	4	5	6	7	8	9	10

Location	**Weather**
	Other symptoms

Triggers

Details

Relief solutions

Medication

Other

Notes

Headache Log

DATE	TIME STARTED
DURATION	TIME ENDED

Severity of headache

0	1	2	3	4	5	6	7	8	9	10

LOCATION	WEATHER
	OTHER SYMPTOMS

Triggers

DETAILS

Relief solutions

MEDICATION

OTHER

NOTES

Headache Log

DATE	TIME STARTED
DURATION	TIME ENDED

Severity of headache

0	1	2	3	4	5	6	7	8	9	10

LOCATION	WEATHER
	OTHER SYMPTOMS

Triggers

DETAILS

Relief solutions

MEDICATION

OTHER

NOTES

Headache Log

DATE	TIME STARTED
DURATION	TIME ENDED

Severity of headache

| 0 | 1 | 2 | 3 | 4 | 5 | 6 | 7 | 8 | 9 | 10 |

LOCATION	WEATHER
	OTHER SYMPTOMS

Triggers

DETAILS

Relief solutions

MEDICATION

OTHER

NOTES

Headache Log

DATE	TIME STARTED
DURATION	TIME ENDED

Severity of headache

0	1	2	3	4	5	6	7	8	9	10

LOCATION	WEATHER
	OTHER SYMPTOMS

Triggers

DETAILS

Relief solutions

MEDICATION

OTHER

NOTES

Headache Log

DATE	TIME STARTED
DURATION	TIME ENDED

Severity of headache

0	1	2	3	4	5	6	7	8	9	10

LOCATION	WEATHER
	OTHER SYMPTOMS

Triggers

DETAILS

Relief solutions

MEDICATION

OTHER

NOTES

Headache Log

DATE	TIME STARTED
DURATION	TIME ENDED

Severity of headache

0 1 2 3 4 5 6 7 8 9 10

LOCATION	WEATHER
	OTHER SYMPTOMS

Triggers

DETAILS

Relief solutions

MEDICATION

OTHER

NOTES

Headache Log

DATE	TIME STARTED
DURATION	TIME ENDED

Severity of headache

| 0 | 1 | 2 | 3 | 4 | 5 | 6 | 7 | 8 | 9 | 10 |

LOCATION	WEATHER
	OTHER SYMPTOMS

Triggers

DETAILS

Relief solutions

MEDICATION

OTHER

NOTES

HEADACHE LOG

DATE	TIME STARTED
DURATION	TIME ENDED

SEVERITY OF HEADACHE

0   1   2   3   4   5   6   7   8   9   10

LOCATION	WEATHER
	OTHER SYMPTOMS

TRIGGERS

DETAILS

RELIEF SOLUTIONS

MEDICATION

OTHER

NOTES

Headache Log

DATE	TIME STARTED
DURATION	TIME ENDED

Severity of headache

0	1	2	3	4	5	6	7	8	9	10

LOCATION	WEATHER
	OTHER SYMPTOMS

Triggers

DETAILS

Relief solutions

MEDICATION

OTHER

NOTES

Headache Log

DATE	**TIME STARTED**
DURATION	**TIME ENDED**

SEVERITY OF HEADACHE

0   1   2   3   4   5   6   7   8   9   10

LOCATION	**WEATHER**
	OTHER SYMPTOMS

TRIGGERS

DETAILS

RELIEF SOLUTIONS

MEDICATION

OTHER

NOTES

Headache Log

DATE	TIME STARTED
DURATION	TIME ENDED

SEVERITY OF HEADACHE

| 0 | 1 | 2 | 3 | 4 | 5 | 6 | 7 | 8 | 9 | 10 |

LOCATION	WEATHER
	OTHER SYMPTOMS

TRIGGERS

DETAILS

RELIEF SOLUTIONS

MEDICATION

OTHER

NOTES

HEADACHE LOG

DATE		TIME STARTED	
DURATION		**TIME ENDED**	

SEVERITY OF HEADACHE

0	1	2	3	4	5	6	7	8	9	10

LOCATION	WEATHER
	OTHER SYMPTOMS

TRIGGERS

DETAILS

RELIEF SOLUTIONS

MEDICATION

OTHER

NOTES

Headache Log

Date	Time started
Duration	Time ended

Severity of headache

0	1	2	3	4	5	6	7	8	9	10

Location	Weather
	Other symptoms

Triggers

Details

Relief solutions

Medication

Other

Notes

HEADACHE LOG

DATE		TIME STARTED	
DURATION		TIME ENDED	

SEVERITY OF HEADACHE

0	1	2	3	4	5	6	7	8	9	10

LOCATION	WEATHER
	OTHER SYMPTOMS

TRIGGERS

DETAILS

RELIEF SOLUTIONS

MEDICATION

OTHER

NOTES

Headache Log

DATE	TIME STARTED
DURATION	TIME ENDED

Severity of headache

0	1	2	3	4	5	6	7	8	9	10

LOCATION	WEATHER
	OTHER SYMPTOMS

Triggers

DETAILS

Relief solutions

MEDICATION

OTHER

NOTES

Headache Log

DATE	TIME STARTED
DURATION	TIME ENDED

Severity of headache

0	1	2	3	4	5	6	7	8	9	10

LOCATION	WEATHER
	OTHER SYMPTOMS

Triggers

DETAILS

Relief solutions

MEDICATION

OTHER

NOTES

Headache Log

DATE	TIME STARTED
DURATION	TIME ENDED

Severity of headache

0	1	2	3	4	5	6	7	8	9	10

LOCATION	WEATHER
	OTHER SYMPTOMS

Triggers

DETAILS

Relief solutions

MEDICATION

OTHER

NOTES

Headache Log

DATE	TIME STARTED
DURATION	TIME ENDED

Severity of headache

0 1 2 3 4 5 6 7 8 9 10

LOCATION	WEATHER
	OTHER SYMPTOMS

Triggers

DETAILS

Relief solutions

MEDICATION

OTHER

NOTES

HEADACHE LOG

DATE	TIME STARTED
DURATION	TIME ENDED

SEVERITY OF HEADACHE

0 1 2 3 4 5 6 7 8 9 10

LOCATION	WEATHER
	OTHER SYMPTOMS

TRIGGERS

DETAILS

RELIEF SOLUTIONS

MEDICATION

OTHER

NOTES

Headache Log

DATE	TIME STARTED
DURATION	TIME ENDED

Severity of headache

0	1	2	3	4	5	6	7	8	9	10

LOCATION	WEATHER
	OTHER SYMPTOMS

Triggers

DETAILS

Relief solutions

MEDICATION

OTHER

NOTES

Headache Log

DATE	TIME STARTED
DURATION	TIME ENDED

Severity of headache

0	1	2	3	4	5	6	7	8	9	10

LOCATION	WEATHER
	OTHER SYMPTOMS

Triggers

DETAILS

Relief solutions

MEDICATION

OTHER

NOTES

Headache Log

DATE	TIME STARTED
DURATION	TIME ENDED

Severity of headache

0	1	2	3	4	5	6	7	8	9	10

LOCATION	WEATHER
	OTHER SYMPTOMS

Triggers

DETAILS

Relief solutions

MEDICATION

OTHER

NOTES

Headache Log

DATE	TIME STARTED
DURATION	**TIME ENDED**

Severity of headache

0	1	2	3	4	5	6	7	8	9	10

LOCATION	WEATHER
	OTHER SYMPTOMS

Triggers

DETAILS

Relief solutions

MEDICATION

OTHER

NOTES

www.ingramcontent.com/pod-product-compliance
Lightning Source LLC
Chambersburg PA
CBHW051026030426
42336CB00015B/2748